TRAIN YOUR BRAIN:

The surprising truth about how to improve your memory

Table of content

Chapter 1:

Improving your memory

Memory loss is unusual forgetfulness. You may not be able to remember new events, recall one or more memories of the past, or both.

The memory loss may be for a short time and then resolve (transient). Or, it may not go away, and, depending on the cause, it can get worse over time.

In severe cases, such memory impairment may interfere with daily living activities.

The word "memory" describes several interconnected abilities. Those abilities rely on many different areas of your brain working together properly. Memory loss can happen when memory-related brain areas don't work as they should.

Commonly, memory loss is a symptom of other medical conditions. It's also important to know that minor memory difficulties, like taking longer to remember things, are typical as you age.

If it simply takes longer to remember things but your memory still works, it's less likely to be a form of disease. However, if you've experienced something that makes you question if you have memory loss, you're certainly not alone.

Alternative Names

Forgetfulness; Amnesia; Impaired memory; Loss of memory; Amnestic syndrome; Dementia - memory loss; Mild cognitive impairment - memory loss.

What does memory loss look like?

Again, it's important to know that true memory loss isn't just slowed recall. If you can remember things with enough time and without hints, it's probably not memory loss.

Memory loss can often look like the following:
- Asking the same question multiple times.
- Trouble remembering recent conversations.
- Misplacing commonly used items.
- Missing appointments.
- Forgetting to pay bills or handle other responsibilities.

If these symptoms appear with any of the following, it's a good idea to see a healthcare provider:

- Trouble saying or finding the right word (aphasia).
- Having difficulty with tasks you could do previously without issue (apraxia).
- Trouble recognizing things, such as faces or familiar items (agnosia).
- Trouble with impulse control, planning, or concentrating attention (executive dysfunction)

It's also important to note that trouble remembering things can happen when you're tired or having issues with the quality of your sleep. This isn't a memory loss. Your brain just isn't working at its best, and it's struggling to access or form memories.

What are the different types of memory loss?

Memory loss can be acute and happen suddenly. It can also be progressive, meaning it happens repetitively and worsens gradually over time.
- **Acute memory loss**: Commonly known as amnesia, this usually happens because of a sudden illness, injury, or other events that disrupt your memory processes.

- **Progressive memory loss**: This is memory loss that happens gradually. It's sometimes a symptom of a degenerative brain disease.

Causes of memory loss

Normal ageing can cause some forgetfulness. It is normal to have some trouble learning new material or needing more time to remember it. However normal ageing does not lead to dramatic memory loss. Such memory loss is due to other diseases.

Memory loss can be caused by many things. To determine a cause, your healthcare provider will ask if the problem came on suddenly or slowly.

Many areas of the brain help you create and retrieve memories. A problem in any of these areas can lead to memory loss.

Memory loss may result from a new injury to the brain, which is caused by or is present after:

· Brain tumour

· Cancer treatment, such as brain radiation, bone marrow transplant, or chemotherapy

· Concussion or head trauma

· Not enough oxygen getting to the brain when your heart or breathing is stopped for too long

· Severe brain infection or infection around the brain

· Major surgery or severe illness, including brain surgery

· Transient global amnesia (sudden, temporary loss of memory) of unclear cause

· Transient ischemic attack (TIA) or stroke

· Hydrocephalus (fluid collection in the brain)

· Multiple sclerosis

· Dementia

Sometimes, memory loss occurs with mental health problems, such as:

· After a major, traumatic, or stressful event

· Bipolar disorder

· Depression or other mental health disorders, such as schizophrenia

Memory loss may be a sign of dementia. Dementia also affects thinking, language, judgment, and behaviour. Common types of dementia associated with memory loss are:

· Alzheimer disease

· Vascular dementia

· Lewy body dementia

· Fronto-temporal dementia

· Progressive supranuclear palsy

· Normal pressure hydrocephalus

· Creutzfeldt-Jakob disease

Other causes of memory loss include:

· Alcohol or use of prescription or illegal drugs

· Brain infections such as Lyme disease, syphilis, or HIV/AIDS

· Overuse of medicines, such as barbiturates or (hypnotics)

· ECT (electroconvulsive therapy) (most often short-term memory loss)

· Epilepsy that is not well controlled

· Illness that results in the loss of or damage to brain tissue or nerve cells, such as Parkinson's disease, Huntington's disease, or multiple sclerosis

· Low levels of important nutrients or vitamins, such as low vitamin B1 or B12

Chapter 2

Difference between mild cognitive impairment and dementia

When older patients and their families report symptoms of "memory loss," experienced clinicians know that these concerns refer to a range of cognitive abilities or general cognitive decline, and not just memory. However, some degree of cognitive slowing is typical of normal ageing.

The clinician's first challenge, therefore, is to identify the cognitive changes that are clinically significant. **Dementia** is typically diagnosed when acquired cognitive impairment has become severe enough to compromise social and/or occupational functioning.

Mild cognitive impairment (MCI) is a state intermediate between normal cognition and dementia, with essentially preserved functional abilities.

Dementia requires substantial impairment to be present in one or (usually) more cognitive domains. The impairment must be sufficient to interfere with independence in everyday activities.

The diagnosis of Mild Neurocognitive Disorder, corresponding to MCI, is made when there is modest impairment in one or more cognitive domains. The individual is still independent in everyday activities, albeit with greater effort.

The impairment must represent a decline from a previously higher level and should be documented both by history and by objective assessment. Further, the cognitive deficits must not occur exclusively in the context of delirium or be better explained by another mental disorder.

The common reason you have trouble recalling things that are on the "tip of your tongue □

"Oh, I loved that movie! And what's-her-name was great in it. You know that actress with the long, light brown hair. And she played that country singer. Hang on, I know this ..."

Most of us have had a case of "tip of the tongue" syndrome at some point. The phenomenon is so common it has clinical shorthand, a "TOT state." It occurs when the left temporal and frontal areas of your brain temporarily fail to work together to retrieve words or names stored in your memory, or other information, like where you left your keys.

Multitasking, fatigue, and the natural ageing process all contribute to your chances of having a TOT moment, but surprising new research claims a simple trick could help you better retain and recall memories, even under stress.

Those findings, published in the online science journal PLOS ONE, reveal that clenching your right fist can give you a better grip on your memory.

A research team from Montclair State University in New Jersey asked subjects (all of whom were right-handed) to clench their left or right hand immediately before trying to memorise a list of words and again before trying to recall it.

The group that clenched their right fists when memorizing the words and their left fists when remembering them scored better on tests of recall than any other group, including those who didn't clench their fists at all.

"The findings suggest that some simple body movements, by temporarily changing the way the brain functions, can improve memory," lead researcher Ruth Popper said in a statement. She believes hand clenching activates specific brain regions associated with memory formation and enables an individual to form stronger memories.

"Future research will examine whether hand clenching can also improve other forms of cognition, for example, verbal or spatial abilities," she added. In other words, remember where you put your keys.

When Things Get Stuck

Tip-of-the-tongue states are believed to affect the average adult about once a week. While it's more common among older people, researchers note, that's not necessarily a bad thing or a warning sign of cognitive failure.

Experiencing a TOT state while trying to recall information is a sign that the information that remains present in your memory can be retrieved even if it takes more time. It usually happens when you're trying to recall names, titles, or words you don't use frequently.

How to Beat TOT

"People can often come up with the first letter and words associated with the word or phrase they're trying to remember," Racine says. You might know a person's name starts with M, for example, or that she has brown hair or often wears a yellow jacket. Still, you can't call up the name.

But the information you do recall could help you unearth the missing name or fact. "Your brain links together related words and activating the neurons in your brain related to one word can cause some activity in related words," Racine says. She advises circumlocution or talking around the world. "That may help activate a network of words that are all related and help the TOT word pop up," she says.

You can also try to tap into your brain's phonological network — a mass of words stored close together because they sound alike (phone, foam, home). Vocalize the words you think might be similar to or sound like the one you're trying to remember.

If you're fighting to recall a former co-worker's name that you think has one syllable and starts with M, just start saying Mike, Mac, Max, and Mark out loud. You could stimulate the network and aid your search.

Forget About It

The most important tip for getting out of a TOT state, the experts say, is not to panic. You'll compound TOT by feeling anxious or nervous that you can't remember the word. A panicky feeling can send your brain into fight-or-flight mode, leaving it unable to concentrate on recalling what's stuck on the tip of your tongue.

One often-successful trick for remembering information is to put the problem out of your mind. Focusing on the fact that you can't remember the word stresses out your brain and doesn't let areas in your brain return to their normal functioning state. When you let go of the search and start to focus on something else, the word will often pop into your head.

7 types of normal memory problems

It's normal to forget things from time to time, and it's normal to become somewhat more forgetful as you age. But how much forgetfulness is too much? How can you tell whether your memory lapses are normal forgetfulness and within the scope of normal ageing or are a symptom of something more serious?

Healthy people can experience memory loss or memory distortion at any age. Some of these memory flaws become more pronounced with age, but — unless they are extreme and persistent.

They are not considered indicators of Alzheimer's or other memory-impairing illnesses.

Seven normal memory problems

1. Transience

This is the tendency to forget facts or events over time. You are most likely to forget information soon after you learn it. However, memory has a use-it-or-lose-it quality: memories that are called up and used frequently are least likely to be forgotten.

Although transience might seem like a sign of memory weakness, brain scientists regard it as beneficial because it clears the brain of unused memories, making way for newer, more useful ones.

2. Absentmindedness

This type of forgetting occurs when you don't pay close enough attention. You forget where you just put your pen because you didn't focus on where you put it in the first place. You were thinking of something else (or, perhaps, nothing in particular), so your brain didn't encode the information securely. Absent-mindedness also involves forgetting to do something at a prescribed time, like taking your medicine or keeping an appointment.

3. Blocking

Someone asks you a question and the answer is right on the tip of your tongue — you know that you know it, but you just can't think of it. This is perhaps the most familiar example of blocking, the temporary inability to retrieve a memory.

In many cases, the barrier is a memory similar to the one you're looking for, and you retrieve the wrong one. This competing memory is so intrusive that you can't think of the memory you want.

Scientists think that memory blocks become more common with age and that they account for the trouble older people have remembering other people's names. Research shows that people can retrieve about half of the blocked memories within just a minute.

4. Misattribution

Misattribution occurs when you remember something accurately in part, but misattribute some detail, like the time, place, or person involved. Another kind of misattribution occurs when you believe a thought you had was original when, in fact, it came from something you had previously read or heard but had forgotten about.

This sort of misattribution explains cases of unintentional plagiarism, in which a writer passes off some information as original when he or she read it somewhere before.

As with several other kinds of memory lapses, misattribution becomes more common with age. As you age, you absorb fewer details when acquiring information because you have somewhat more trouble concentrating and processing information rapidly. And as you grow older, your memories grow older as well. And old memories are especially prone to misattribution.

5. Suggestibility

Suggestibility is the vulnerability of your memory to the power of suggestion — information that you learn about an occurrence after the fact becomes incorporated into your memory of the incident, even though you did not experience these details.

Although little is known about exactly how suggestibility works in the brain, the suggestion fools your mind into thinking it's a real memory.

6. Bias

Even the sharpest memory isn't a flawless snapshot of reality. In your memory, your perceptions are filtered by your personal biases — experiences, beliefs, prior knowledge, and even your mood at the moment.

Your biases affect your perceptions and experiences when they're being encoded in your brain. And when you retrieve a memory, your mood and other biases at that moment can influence what information you recall.

Although everyone's attitudes and preconceived notions bias their memories, there's been virtually no research on the brain mechanisms behind memory bias or whether it becomes more common with age.

7. Persistence

Most people worry about forgetting things. But in some cases, people are tormented by memories they wish they could forget, but can't. The persistence of memories of traumatic events, negative feelings, and ongoing fears is another form of memory problem.

Some of these memories accurately reflect horrifying events, while others may be negative distortions of reality.

People suffering from depression are particularly prone to having persistent, disturbing memories. So are people with post-traumatic stress disorder (PTSD). PTSD can result from many different forms of traumatic exposure — for example, sexual abuse or wartime experiences. Flashbacks, which are persistent, intrusive memories of the traumatic event, are a core feature of PTSD.

Chapter 3

Why depression can make it harder to forget unpleasant experiences

Depression has been linked to memory problems, such as forgetfulness or confusion. It can also make it difficult to focus on work or other tasks, make decisions, or think clearly. Stress and anxiety can also lead to poor memory.

Depression is associated with short-term memory loss. It doesn't affect other types of memory, such as long-term memory and procedural memory, which control motor skills.

Symptoms of depression may include sadness and changes in mood. However, depression is a complex diagnosis that can affect many aspects of functioning. This can include impacting memory.

While we often associate depression with low mood, tiredness, and feelings of hopelessness, less well-known is that some people with depression may experience problems with their memory – such as feeling more forgetful than usual.

Though memory problems aren't discussed as widely as other symptoms, we know that cognitive impairments are common in depression. Up to three in five people with depression may experience them. It's thought that these memory problems are related to the changes in our brain's structure and function that happen because of depression.

Memory problems can occur when depression first begins and can persist, even when other depressive symptoms have improved. Typically, it's our working memory that's affected. This is the short-term memory we use to actively remember things from moment to moment – and problems with it can make it difficult to concentrate or make decisions. Many cognitive functions are often affected, such as response time, attention and planning, decision-making, and reasoning.

Depression also makes it difficult for our brain to switch between tasks and inhibit what can be knee-jerk responses.

The severity of memory problems can vary from person to person. However, some research shows cognitive impairments tend to be smaller in the first episode of depression, while worse memory problems have been seen with more severe depressive symptoms and repeated episodes of low mood.

These effects on memory can even last when there are few or no symptoms of depression.

Brain structure and function

Depression is linked to widespread changes in brain structure and function – including in the prefrontal cortex, hippocampus, and amygdala. These regions are all involved in cognition, executive function (such as planning, decision-making, and reasoning), and emotion processing.

These regions are interlinked via neural circuits, and they send and receive messages from each other, so problems in one region will impact on others. And, the neural circuits responsible for cognition and emotion processing overlap with those that control our stress response systems. So periods of high stress can also impair cognitive function and worsen mood.

The changes in these brain regions seen in depression can have a big impact on how well our brain works during memory tasks.

For example, people with depression often have a smaller hippocampus and have increased activity extending from the prefrontal cortex during a working memory task in which they were asked to remember specific letters.

This meant the brains of people with depression had to work harder during the memory task by recruiting the help of additional brain regions to perform at the same level as participants who didn't have depression.

The circuits that connect cognition (including memory) and emotion use chemical messengers – such as serotonin, dopamine, noradrenaline, and glutamate – which allow neurons in these brain regions to communicate with each other.

Since brain messenger systems are continually interacting with each other, changes within them mean our neurons may be less able to communicate with each other. This may also affect how our memory works.

Working memory

This isn't to say there aren't still many things a person struggling with depression can do to improve their memory.

For example, exercise is shown to benefit working memory, processing speed, and attention. Its thought that exercises releases brain messengers (including serotonin and dopamine) and increases activation in the brain's cortex.

These both increase the growth of new neurons and brain plasticity (the brain's ability to change, adapt and grow). All of this is important for good memory.

Talking therapies also show increased activation in the prefrontal cortex, which could be linked with improved responsiveness and flexibility, both important aspects of cognition and mood. Cognitive training programs – such as cognitive exercises or games, usually done on a computer – can even improve working memory and attention.

In some cases, antidepressants can help to improve working memory.

The most commonly prescribed antidepressants, selective serotonin reuptake inhibitors (SSRI) and serotonergic-noradrenergic reuptake inhibitors (SNRI) are also associated with improvements in planning, decision-making, and reasoning – though these findings are mixed, and may not work as well for older people. Novel brain stimulation treatments, which affect how neurons can send signals, have also been associated with improvements in cognitive functions.

Memory problems can be a common symptom of depression and can have a serious impact on our day-to-day lives, including how well we perform at work and our relationships with other people.

This is why it's important to consider memory problems alongside other core symptoms of depression – such as low mood – to improve treatment and prevent recurrence.

Chapter 4

How to manage memory loss

Very little research has evaluated strategies for treating memory loss in people with depression. For some people, treating depression may ease memory loss. A healthcare provider can help a person compare treatment options and track changes over time.

There are various ways a person can help to improve their memory. These include exercise, meditation, and getting adequate sleep.

Most people have occasional lapses in memory, such as forgetting a new acquaintance's name or misplacing the car keys. Most of the time, this is simply a sign that a person is a bit too busy or preoccupied. On the other hand, having a consistently poor memory can be problematic for someone.

Many factors play a role in memory loss, including genetics, age, and medical conditions that affect the brain. There are also some manageable risk factors for memory loss, such as diet and lifestyle.

While not all memory loss is preventable, people may be able to take measures to protect the brain against cognitive decline as they age.

In this article, learn about eight techniques to try to help improve your memory.

1. Do brain training

In a similar way to muscles, the brain needs regular use to stay healthy. Mental workouts are just as essential to grey matter as other factors, and challenging the mind can help it grow and expand, which may improve memory.

A large trial from the journal *PLoS One* Trusted Source found that people who did just 15 minutes of brain training activities at least 5 days a week had improvements in brain function.

The participants' working memory, short-term memory, and problem-solving skills all significantly improved when researchers compared them to a control group doing crossword puzzles.

The researchers used brain training activities from the website Lumosity. The challenges work on a person's ability to recall details and quickly memorise patterns.

2. Exercise

Physical exercise has a direct impact on brain health. Regular exercise reduces the risk of cognitive decline with age and protects the brain against degeneration.

The results of research suggest that aerobic exercise can improve memory function in people with early Alzheimer's disease. The control group did anaerobic stretching and toning.

Aerobic exercise increases a person's heart rate and can include any of these activities:

- brisk walking
- running
- hiking
- swimming
- dancing
- cross-country skiing

3. Meditate

Mindfulness meditation may help improve memory. Note that many studies show meditation improves brain function, reduces markers of brain degeneration, and improves both working memory and long-term memory.

The researchers observed the brains of people who regularly practised meditation and those who did not.

Their results indicated that making a habit of meditating may cause long-term changes in the brain, including increasing brain plasticity, which helps keep it healthy.

4. Get enough sleep

Sleep is vital for overall brain health. Disrupting the body's natural sleep cycle can lead to cognitive impairments, as this interrupts the processes the brain uses to create memories.

Getting a full night's rest, typically about 7 to 9 hours a night for an adult, helps the brain create and store long-term memories.

5. Reduce sugar intake

Sugary foods can taste delicious and feel rewarding at first, but they may play a role in memory loss. A diet high in sugary drinks has a link to Alzheimer's disease.

Also drinking too many sugary drinks, including fruit juice, may have a connection to a lower total brain volume, which is an early sign of Alzheimer's disease.

Avoiding extra sugar may help combat this risk. While naturally sweet foods, such as fruits, are a good addition to a healthful diet, people can avoid drinks sweetened with sugar and foods with added, processed sugars.

6. Avoid high-calorie diets

Along with cutting out sources of excess sugar, reducing overall caloric intake may also help protect the brain.

High-calorie diets can impair memory and lead to obesity. The effects on memory may be due to how high-calorie diets lead to inflammation in particular parts of the brain.

While most research in this area has been with animals, a study from 2009 looked at whether restricting calories in humans could improve memory.

Female participants with an average age of 60.5 years reduced their calorie intake by 30%. The researchers found that they had a significant improvement in verbal memory scores and that the benefit was most significant in those who stuck to the diet best.

Other strategies may also help. Those include:

- creating reminders for upcoming events
- slowing down to commit information to memory
- working in a distraction-free environment where possible
- focusing on one thing at a time
- using digital calendars for automatic notifications

Many techniques for improving memory can be beneficial for a person's overall health and well-being. For example, practicing mindfulness meditation may not only make a person less forgetful but can also reduce stress.

Even adding one or two memory-boosting practices to a person's daily routine may help them keep their brain healthy and protect it from memory loss.

Chapter 5

Strategies used to make new information stick like a long-term memory

Memories may serve as fond reminders of the past, but they also allow us to achieve learning goals and expand our educational horizons in the here and now. It would be nice if our minds functioned like cameras and we could access our picture-like memories at any time we wanted. Unfortunately, this is not how it works; everything we see and hear is stored in different areas of our brains and we can easily lose information if we don't make a conscious effort to retain it. In this article, I'll explore the basics of long-term memory and I'll share a few strategies that can help you.

The Long-Term Memory Types

Many cognitive psychologists believe that long-term memory is divided into two distinct types: explicit memory and implicit memory.

1. **Explicit or Declarative Memory.**

Explicit memory, also known as declarative memory, is made up of memories that we are conscious of remembering and capable of describing in words. Explicit memory can be subdivided into semantic memory, which refers to our memories that are drawn from common knowledge, such as facts and general knowledge about the world, for example, the names of colours, and episodic memory, which refers to memories that are drawn from our personal experiences.

2. **Implicit or Nondeclarative Memory.**

Implicit memory, also known as non-declarative memory, consists of subconscious memories, like knowledge that allow us to carry out basic tasks without even realizing we are recalling the information. For example, when you type on a keyboard you are not conscious of the long-term memories that are allowing you to perform the function.

Information that is encoded in implicit memory, such as knowledge concerning our body movements, can be recalled automatically, without us needing to make a conscious effort. Because it flows effortlessly in our actions, it is often difficult to be verbalized, that's why it's also known as "non-declarative".

Implicit memory can also be subdivided into two types: procedural, which refers to recalling how to do things that require action, such as walking or playing the piano and priming memory, which refers to the automatic activation of certain associations of new with previous knowledge.

A popular example that describes how priming memory works is that when one reads the word "yellow", they will recognize the word "banana" slightly faster than the word "sea".

Cognitive Processes Involved In The Long-Term Memory

Long-term memory is not just a permanent storage that archives information. It also involves another cognitive mechanism such as providing the working memory with relevant background information for the latter to acquire meaning. The long-term memory, therefore, performs three basic operations: encoding, storage, and retrieval.

1. **Encoding.**

Encoding is the ability to convert data we collect into a knowledge-based structure known as schemata. New information is either just added to existing schemata enriching them, or contradicts with them and finally manages to alter them. The first process is known as assimilation, though the second is accommodation.

2. **Storage.**

Simply put, storage is the ability of long-term memory to store information in different brain areas. For example, semantic memories, such as facts are stored in different brain areas than automating procedural memories, such as how to ride a bike. We cannot be sure, neither for how long, nor for how much information can be stored in the long-term memory.

Theoretically speaking, long-term memory has unlimited capacity, and information there can be stored for the rest of our lives. It is also still debatable whether information stored in long-term memory can be permanently deleted, as "deletion" may involve just the inability to locate or retrieve information, rather than permanent loss.

It has been found that **<u>forgetting</u>** is the result of either poor initial encoding of information or poor retrieval methods.

3.   **Retrieval.**

Retrieval, or else, remembering. Retrieval of information is the process of not only activating but also using information that is stored in long-term memory.

There are two distinct forms of retrieval: recall, which refers to generating or reproducing stored information we've already acquired, and recognition, which refers to identifying stored information that is familiar.

Needless to say, recognition is much more effective than recall, as meaningful associations don't require as much depth of processing or cognitive effort.

Enhancing Long-Term Memory

Indeed, it is quite challenging to find how to process information in ways that will keep it fresh and accessible. But I believe these strategies will be of great help.

Start with mnemonic devices

Mnemonic devices are learning strategies used to boost your memory. Whether or not you realize it, you probably use mnemonics in your daily life to help you retain and recall information. I'll start with some of the most common mnemonic devices before moving on to other memorization tactics.

1. Acronyms and acrostics

You may already be familiar with acronyms and acrostics as a mnemonic device. This method requires you to create a new word or group of words by taking the first letter of each word and putting them together.

For example, to remember the names of the planets in our solar system, you might use this acrostic mnemonic: **my v**ery **e**ducated **m**other **j**ust **s**erved **us noodles**. In this example, the first letter of each word corresponds with the first letter of each planet, respectively.

2. Music mnemonics

My partner knows all the words to House of Pain's *Jump Around*—yet he can't remember what I asked him to pick up from the grocery store an hour ago.

Why? Because it's easier to remember a catchy song than it is to remember a long string of meaningless words or letters, such as a grocery list yelled to you while you're halfway out the door.

The next time you need to remember something, try pairing that information with a tune you're already familiar with. And if you just so happen to need help memorizing the periodic table of elements, look no further than the periodic table song.

3. Create a memory palace

The memory palace technique, also known as the Method of Loci, is another popular mnemonic device.

This technique involves mentally mapping out a physical space you're familiar with (a memory palace) and "placing" images representing the information you're memorizing in various spots or *loci*. (*Loci* is the plural form of *locus*, which means "place" or "location.")

When you need to recall that information, simply visualize your memory palace and retrieve it.

Chapter 6

How to create and use your memory palace

1.   **Choose your memory palace.** Select a space that you're incredibly familiar with (e.g., your childhood home or the route you take to work), and create a mental map of it.

2.   **Identify distinct *loci* throughout your palace.** Mentally walk through your palace, and pick different locations where you can "place" unique images (more on that in step 3). For example, the door to your coat closet, the lamp in your living room, and the dog bed in your guest room.

3.   **Assign images to specific locations.** Let's say you're trying to remember this grocery list: milk, chocolate chip cookies, and bananas. Place images of each of those items at your chosen locations. Or, to make it more memorable, create vivid images representing each item and place those at different locations.

The more animated and outrageous, the better.

For example, you could picture a waterfall of milk pouring over your closet door, your living room lamp teetering on top of a mountain of chocolate chip cookies, and a dog juggling banana while standing on its bed.

While this technique may sound absurd, it *does* work. Just take it from five-time USA Memory Champion Nelson Dellis, who uses the memory palace technique to help him quickly remember a full deck of cards, in sequence.

4.   **Repeat, repeat, repeat.**

Fascinating brain fact: We have 100.000.000.000 (one hundred billion!) neurons in our brain and each of them is connected to 1000 others. Neurons' main role is to transfer information by "firing" impulse signals to their neighbours, who transfer the same signals to other "neighbours" of theirs, and so on.

It's exactly like a domino effect.

The connection between two neurons is called a "synapse" and it increasingly gets stronger, the more frequent the signals between two neurons become.

Because memories, just like thoughts, are represented by the resulting patterns of neuron firing, the stronger the synapse between two neurons, the more reinforced a trace of memory becomes and the higher the likelihood of being retrieved.

5. Use multiple ways to present the information.

Repetition allows you to soak up the information more rapidly and for longer periods, even concepts that may be more difficult to understand. However, it's important to switch up the formats in which the information is delivered.

6. Write it down

While typing your notes might be faster and more convenient, especially if you have to take in a lot of information, there are advantages to doing things the old-fashioned way (i.e., taking pen to paper).

In a 2014 study, researchers Pam A. Mueller and Daniel M. Oppenheimer examined the effects on learning and retention when students took notes by hand versus on a laptop. In terms of generative note-taking (e.g., "summarizing, paraphrasing, concept mapping"), students who took notes by hand had better retention and understanding of the material compared to those who took notes on a laptop.

Why? The researchers suggest two possible reasons. First, there are fewer possible distractions, such as checking emails or social media, when writing notes. Second, generative note-taking encourages students to reframe the information into their own words, which aids in encoding.

Bonus: offload the stuff you *don't* need to memorise

Adult human brains can store the equivalent of 2.5 million gigabytes of memory. So, in theory, you can memorise…everything. But just because you can, doesn't mean you have to.

Instead, use the memorization techniques listed in this article to help you recall the information that you might need at the drop of a hat, like your emergency contact's phone number. Or the password to your password manager. Everything else? Use a note-taking app to take a cognitive load off.

When to get help for memory loss

If you're worried about memory loss, make an appointment with your healthcare provider.

If memory loss affects your ability to do your daily activities, if you notice your memory getting worse, or if a family member or friend is concerned about your memory loss, it's particularly important to get help.

At your appointment, your provider likely will do a physical exam and check your memory and problem-solving skills. Sometimes other tests may be needed too. Treatment depends on what's causing memory loss.